The Drug Awareness Library™

Danger:
CAFFEINE

Patra McSharry Sevastiades

The Rosen Publishing Group's
PowerKids Press™
New York

The people pictured in this book are only models. They in no way practice or endorse the activities illustrated. Captions serve only to explain the subjects of the photographs and do not in any way imply a connection between the real-life models and the staged situations.

Published in 1997 by The Rosen Publishing Group, Inc.
29 East 21st Street, New York, NY 10010

Copyright © 1997 by The Rosen Publishing Group, Inc.

First Edition

Book Design: Erin McKenna

Photo Illustrations: Cover and photo illustrations by Carrie Ann Grippo.

Sevastiades, Patra McSharry.
    Danger: caffeine / Patra McSharry Sevastiades.
        p.   cm. — (The drug awareness library)
    Summary: Explains how caffeine affects the body and the harm overuse of it can cause.
    ISBN 0-8239-5046-8
    1. Caffeine habit—Juvenile literature. 2. Caffeine—Juvenile literature. [1. Caffeine. 2. Drug abuse.] I. Title. II. Series.
    RC567.5.S48   1996
    615'.785—dc20
                                                                            96-44289
                                                                                CIP
                                                                                 AC

Manufactured in the United States of America

Contents

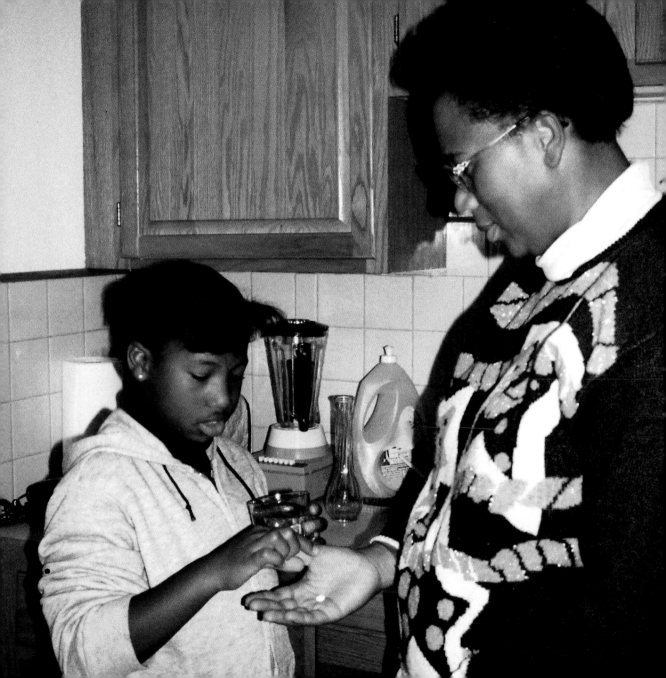

What Are Drugs?

Drugs are things that people use that change the way they feel, think, or act. Some drugs, called medicine, help your body when you are sick. Your parents or your doctor may give you medicine when you don't feel well.

Other drugs can hurt the people who use them. **Caffeine** (kaf-EEN) is one of these drugs.

◀ Medicine helps you get well when you are sick.

What Is Caffeine?

Caffeine comes from many different sources: coffee beans, tea leaves, cocoa beans, and **kola nuts** (KO-la nutz). Caffeine does not have a smell. It tastes bitter.

Caffeine is a **stimulant** (STIM-yoo-lent). That means that it speeds up your body. If someone feels tired and she drinks a cup of coffee with caffeine in it, she will feel more awake for a little while.

Many people drink coffee or tea in the morning to help them wake up. ▶

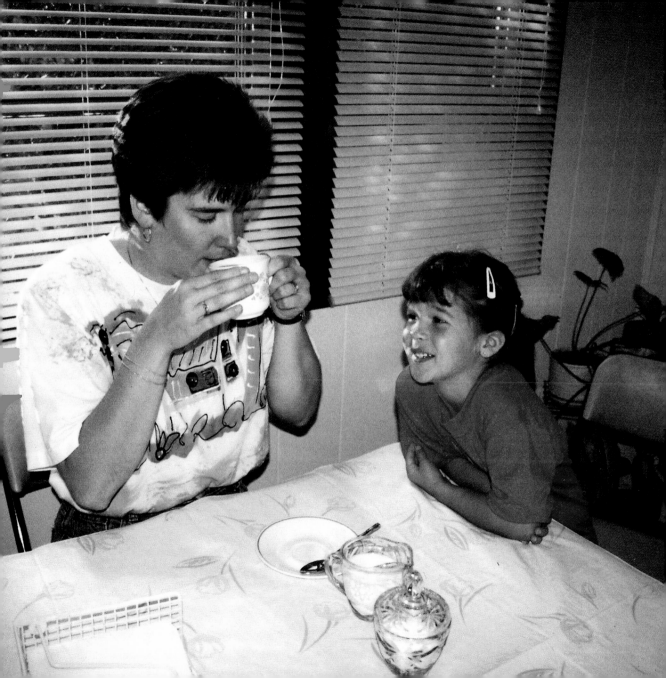

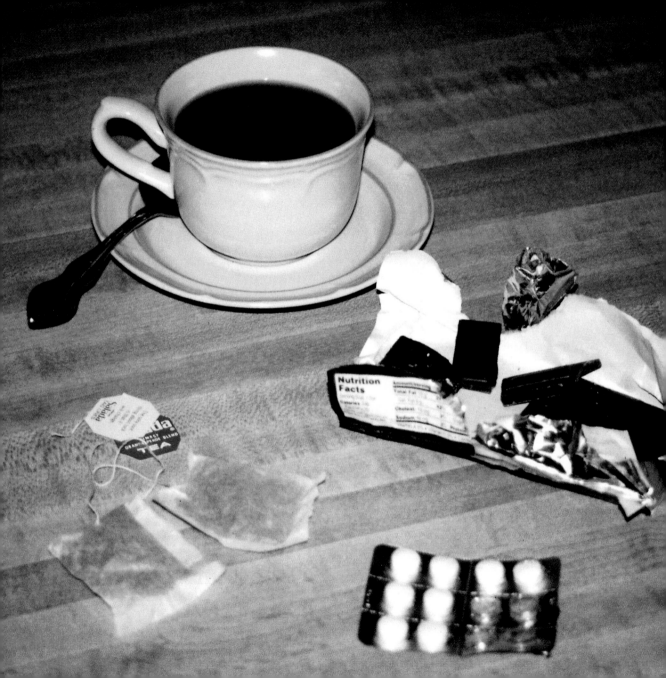

Caffeine Is a Legal Drug

Caffeine is a **legal** (LEE-gul) drug. Even though it can hurt you, many foods contain it. But our **government** (GUV-ern-ment) makes sure that there is not too much caffeine in any product.

Many people do not like what caffeine does to them. Some of these people drink **decaffeinated** (dee-KAF-in-ay-ted) coffee and soft drinks. Others drink decaffeinated tea or **herbal** (UR-bul) tea.

◀ Caffeine is found in many things.

Who Uses Caffeine?

Caffeine is used by people all over the world. Many people eat and drink caffeine every day. It is found in some foods and drinks. In some places, people eat raw coffee beans. You may like to drink a soft drink that has caffeine in it. Your parents may drink tea or coffee that has caffeine in it. If you eat chocolate, you eat caffeine. If you drink hot cocoa, you drink caffeine. It is okay to have a little caffeine. But it hurts your body if you have too much caffeine.

Many people eat or drink caffeine ▶
without even realizing it.

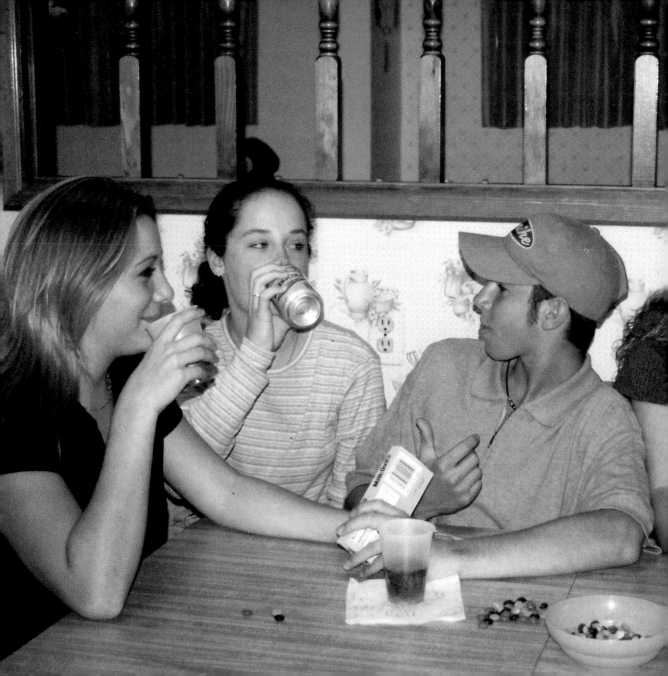

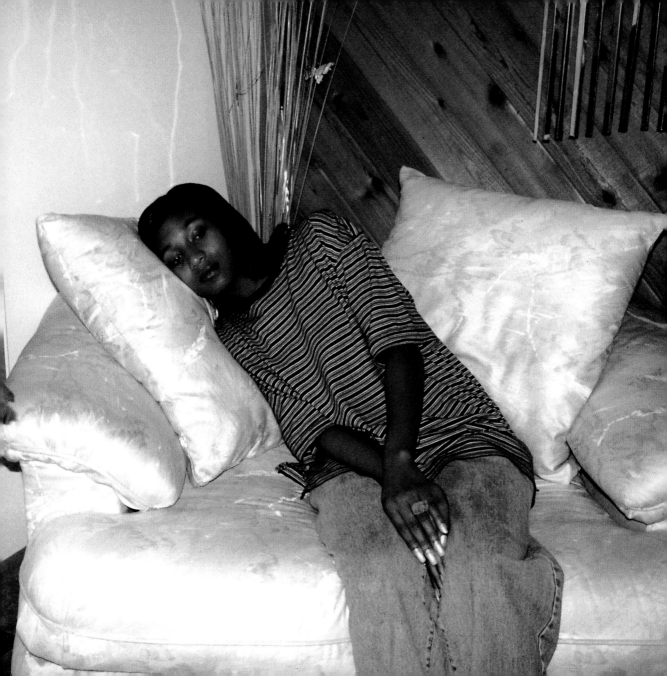

What Does Caffeine Do?

However someone takes caffeine, it ends up in his or her **bloodstream** (BLUD-streem). It travels through the bloodstream to the brain. It makes the heart beat faster. It can cause **blood vessels** (BLUD VESS-elz) to become smaller. That makes it harder for a person's heart to pump blood through his or her body. Caffeine makes a person feel more **alert** (uh-LERT). But a little while later, when the caffeine wears off, that person feels very tired.

◀ A person may feel even more tired when the caffeine wears off.

Caffeine Can Hurt You

Caffeine speeds up your heart. Some people who use caffeine feel **anxious** (ANK-shus) or **irritable** (EER-it-uh-bul). It gives other people stomach problems. Caffeine can also make it harder for people to sleep. This can happen even many hours after a person has something with caffeine in it. And people who use a lot of caffeine usually do not sleep as well as people who do not use it. Some people are **allergic** (uh-LER-jik) to caffeine. Even a little caffeine makes them feel sick.

Some people have trouble falling asleep if they have caffeine before bedtime. ▶

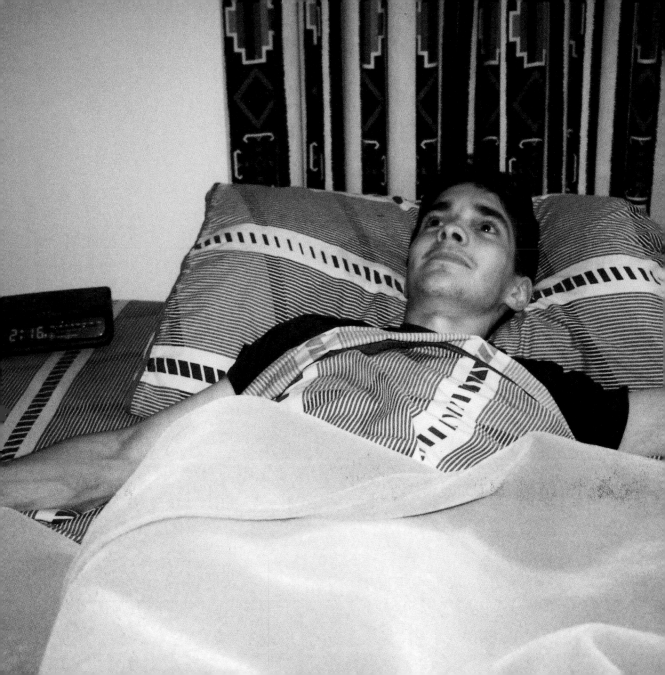

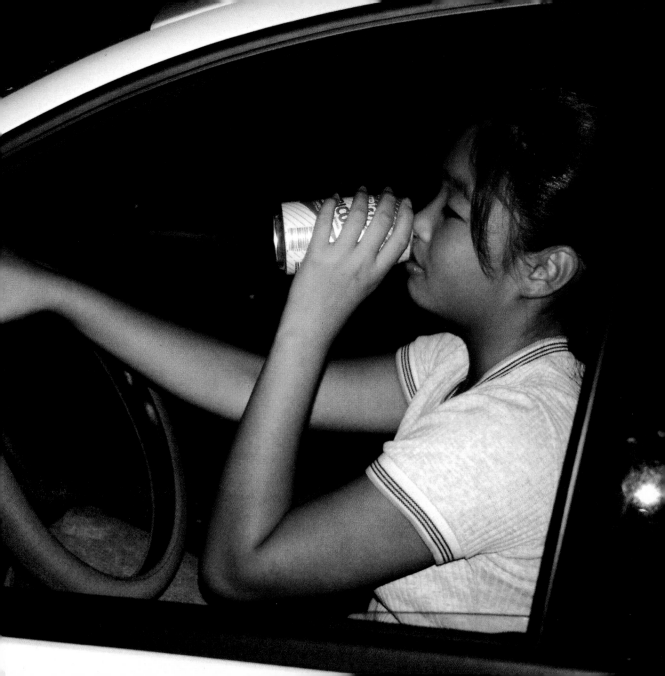

Why People Use Caffeine

Most people use caffeine because they like the taste of soft drinks and the way caffeine makes them feel "up." Or they like the "lift" coffee or tea gives them in the morning. Other people use caffeine to stay awake when they are tired. They may have to drive on a long trip. Or they may want to stay up late to study for a test. But the best thing to do if you are tired is to sleep. You will feel better and more alert if you don't use caffeine.

◀ Sometimes people use caffeine to stay awake.

17

Building Up a Tolerance

If you use caffeine often, your body builds up a **tolerance** (TOL-er-ents) to it. That means that your body gets used to caffeine. Someone who has built up a tolerance to caffeine needs more of it to feel awake. Two cans of soda may not be enough to give a person the lift she wants. She may need to drink three or four cans. Then she may feel jittery or anxious. If someone stops using caffeine, she may have a headache and she may feel tired or sad for a little while.

The more caffeine a person drinks, the more she needs to feel the affects of it. ▶

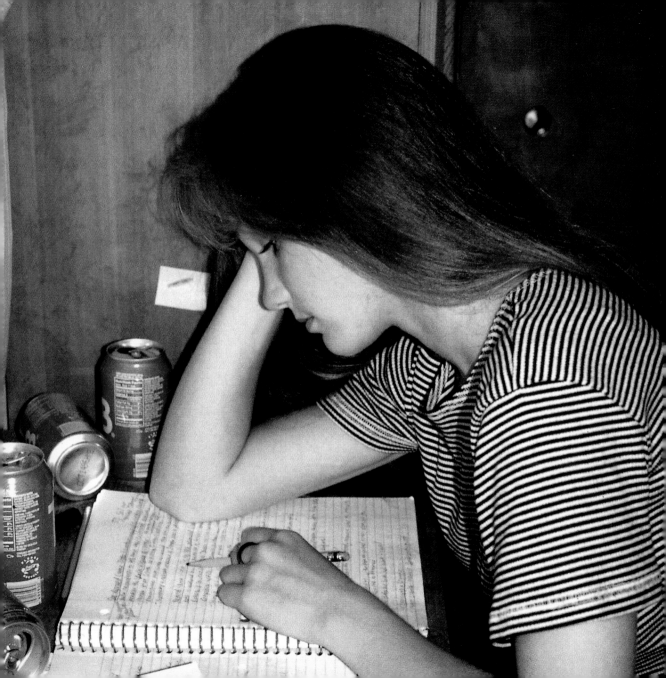

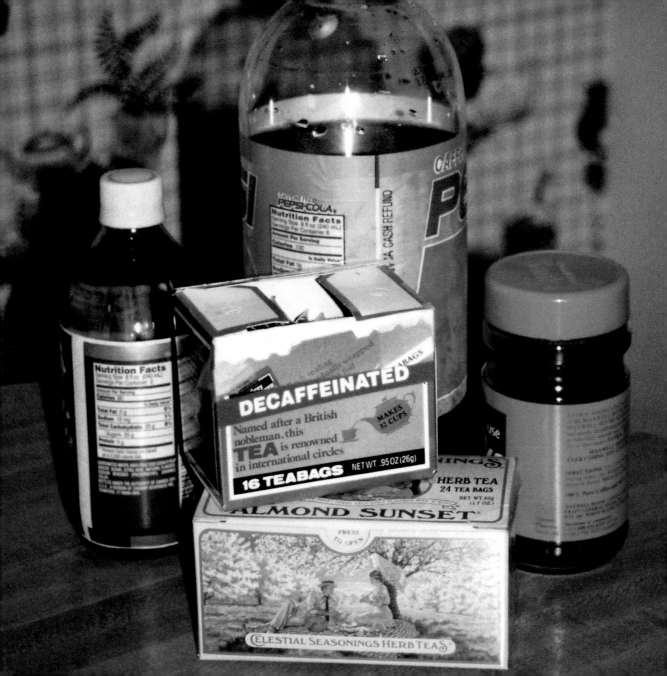

Being Careful

It's okay to drink soft drinks with caffeine every once in a while. It's okay to have chocolate and cocoa sometimes, too. Drinking a cup of coffee or tea once in a while will not hurt someone. But having too much caffeine can hurt your body. It can also keep you from getting the sleep you need.

◀ You and your family may decide to use products that don't have caffeine in them.

Taking Care of Your Body

It's up to you to make sure that you give your body what it needs. This means sleeping when you are tired. It also means being aware of how much caffeine you put into your body. Too much caffeine can hurt you.

One way you can avoid caffeine is to choose drinks that don't have caffeine in them. If you eat sweets, try not to eat too much chocolate. And don't ever take caffeine pills.

Be smart. Take good care of your body.

Glossary

alert (uh-LERT) Wide awake.

allergic (uh-LER-jik) When someone has a bad reaction to a usually harmless thing.

anxious (ANK-shus) Fearful; nervous.

bloodstream (BLUD-streem) The blood flowing through your body.

blood vessel (BLUD VESS-el) A tube in the body through which blood flows.

caffeine (kaf-EEN) A drug that is a stimulant.

decaffeinated (dee-KAF-in-ay-ted) Having no caffeine.

government (GUV-ern-ment) The people who rule a country.

herbal (UR-bul) Made from plants.

irritable (EER-it-uh-bul) Being easily upset.

kola nut (KO-la nut) Seeds of the kola tree.

legal (LEE-gul) Allowed by the law.

stimulant (STIM-yoo-lent) Something that speeds up parts of the body.

tolerance (TOL-er-ents) Needing more of a drug to feel the drug's effects.

23

Index